Dash Diet Cookbook for Beginners

50 Delicacies very Easy to Prepare to Stay fit and enjoy your diet plan in the best possible way

Natalie Puckett

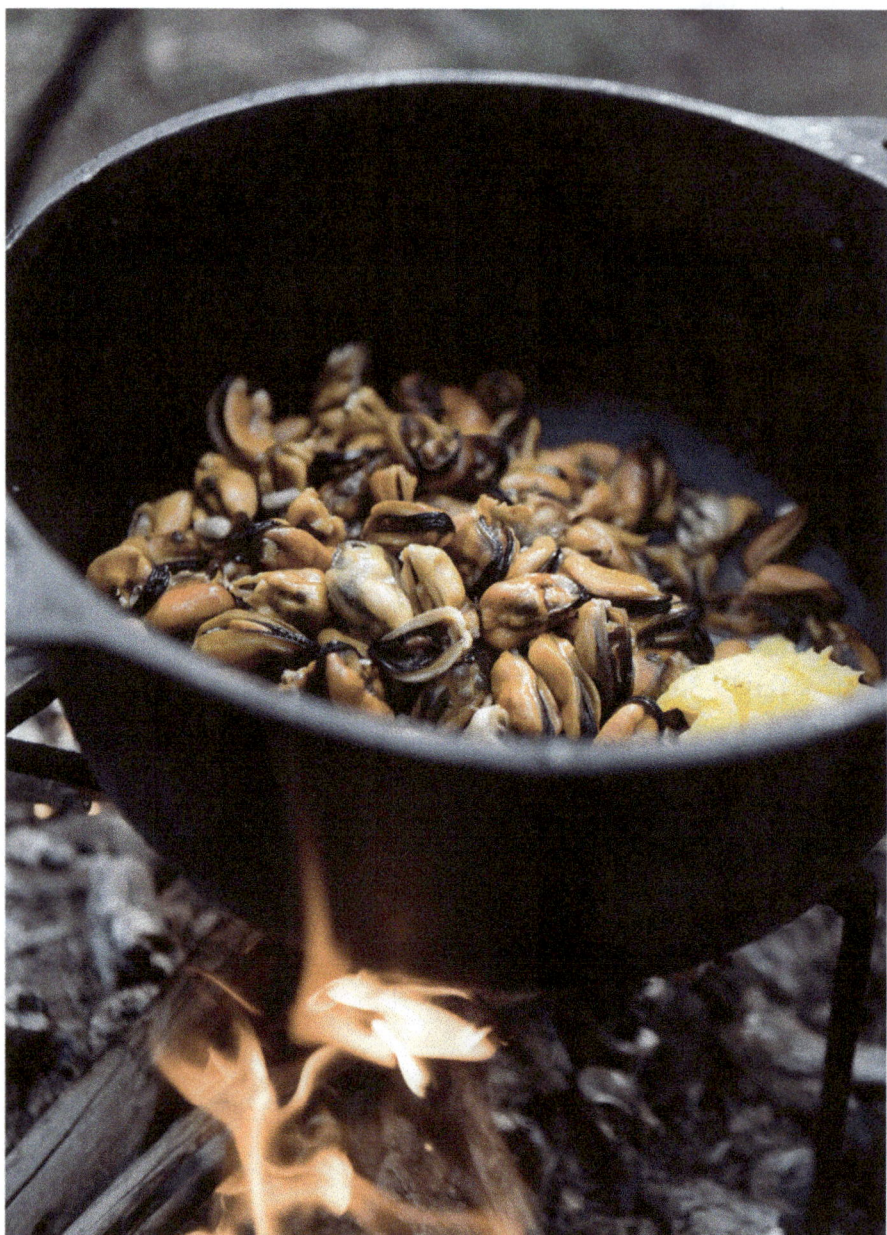

Table of Contents

Simple One Pot Mussels

Serving: 4

Prep Time: 10 minutes

Cook Time: 5 minutes

Ingredients:

2 tablespoons butter

2 chopped shallots

minced garlic cloves

½ cup broth

½ cup white wine

2 pounds cleaned mussels

Lemon and parsley for serving

How To:

1.   Clean the mussels and take away the beard.

2.   Discard any mussels that don't close when tapped against a tough surface.

3.   Set your pot to Sauté mode and add chopped onion and butter.

4. Stir and sauté onions.

5. Add garlic and cook for 1 minute.

6. Add broth and wine.

7. Lock the lid and cook for five minutes on high.

8. Release the pressure naturally over 10 minutes.

9. Serve with a sprinkle of parsley and enjoy!

Nutrition (Per Serving)

Calories: 286

Fats: 14g

Carbs: 12g

Protein: 28g

Lemon Pepper and Salmon

Serving: 3

Prep Time: 5 minutes

Cook Time: 6 minutes

Ingredients:

¾ cup water

Few sprigs of parsley, basil, tarragon, basil 1 pound of salmon, skin on

teaspoons ghee

¼ teaspoon salt

½ teaspoon pepper

½ lemon, thinly sliced

1 whole carrot, julienned

How To:

1.   Set your pot to Sauté mode and water and herbs.

2.   Place a steamer rack inside your pot and place salmon.

3.   Drizzle the ghee on top of the salmon and season with salt and pepper.

4. Cover lemon slices.

5. Lock the lid and cook on high for 3 minutes.

6. Release the pressure naturally over 10 minutes.

7. Transfer the salmon to a serving platter.

8. Set your pot to Sauté mode and add vegetables.

9. Cook for 1-2 minutes.

10. Serve with vegetables and salmon.

11. Enjoy!

Nutrition (Per Serving)

Calories: 464

Fat: 34g

Carbohydrates: 3g

Protein: 34g

Simple Sautéed Garlic and Parsley Scallops

Serving: 4

Prep Time: 5 minutes

Cook Time: 25 minutes

Ingredients:

8 tablespoons almond butter

2 garlic cloves, minced

16 large sea scallops

Sunflower seeds and pepper to taste

1 ½ tablespoons olive oil

How To:

1.   Seasons scallops with sunflower seeds and pepper.

2.   Take a skillet, place it over medium heat, add oil and let it heat up.

3.   Sauté scallops for two minutes per side, repeat until all scallops are cooked.

4.   Add almond butter to the skillet and let it melt.

5.   Stir in garlic and cook for quarter-hour.

6.   Return scallops to skillet and stir to coat.

7.   Serve and enjoy!

Nutrition (Per Serving)

Calories: 417

Fat: 31g

Net Carbohydrates: 5g

Protein: 29g

Salmon and Cucumber Platter

Serving: 4

Prep Time: 10 minutes

Cook Time: nil

Ingredients:

2 cucumbers, cubed

2 teaspoons fresh squeezed lemon juice ounces non-fat yogurt teaspoon lemon zest, grated

Pepper to taste

teaspoons dill, chopped

8 ounces smoked salmon, flaked

How To:

1. Take a bowl and add cucumbers, juice, lemon peel, pepper, dill, salmon, yogurt and toss well.

2.   Serve cold.

3.   Enjoy!

Nutrition (Per Serving)

Calories: 242

Fat: 3g

Carbohydrates: 3g

Protein: 3g

Tuna Paté

Serving: 4

Prep Time: 10 minutes

Cook Time: nil

Ingredients:

ounces canned tuna, drained and flaked teaspoons fresh lemon juice 1 teaspoon onion, minced

ounces low-fat cream cheese

¼ cup parsley, chopped

How To:

1. Take a bowl and blend in tuna, cheese, juice, parsley, onion and stir well.

2. Serve cold and enjoy!

Nutrition (Per Serving)

Calories: 172

Fat: 2g

Carbohydrates: 8g

Protein: 4g

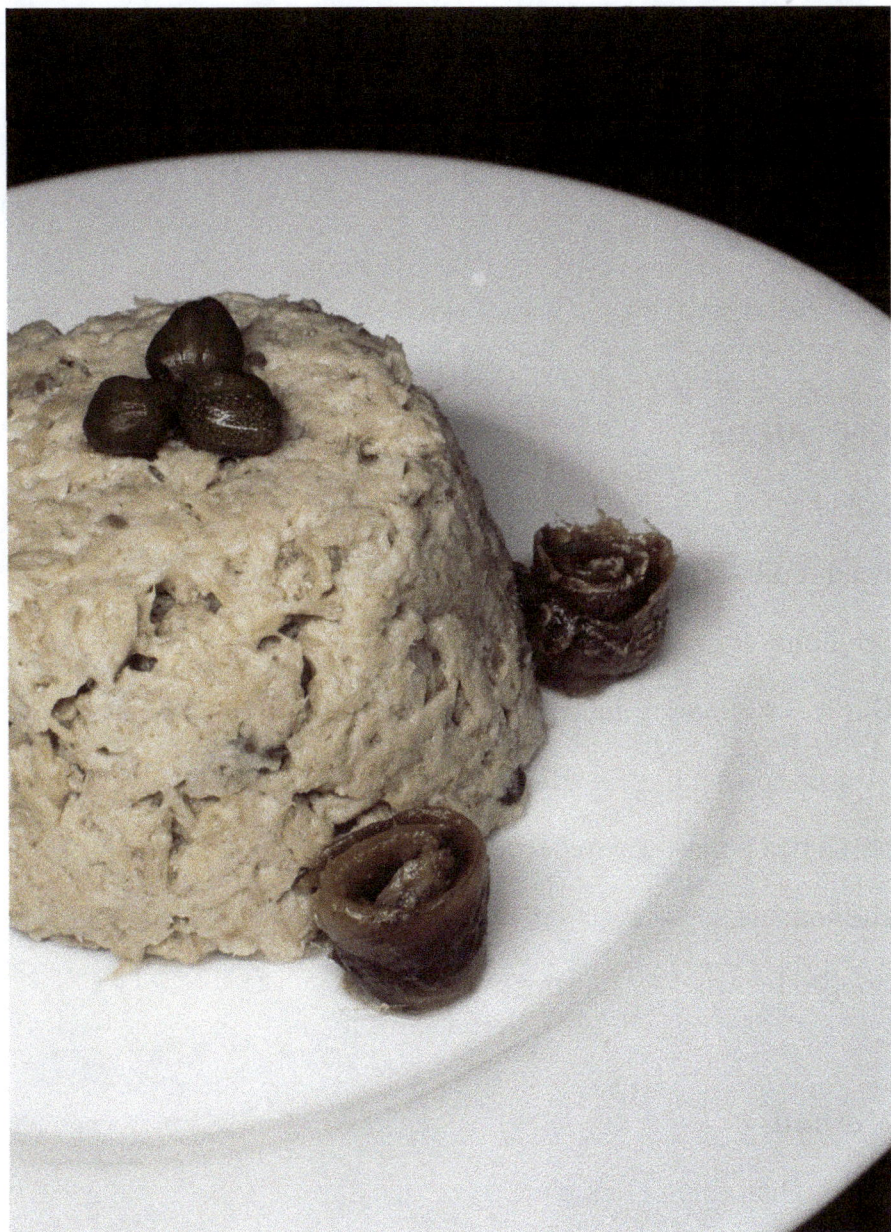

Beef with Pea Pods

Prep time: 5 minutes

Cook time: 10 minutes

Servings: 4

Ingredients

Thin beef steak – ¾ pound, sliced into thin strips

Peanut oil – 1 Tbsp.

Scallions – 3, sliced

Garlic – 2 cloves, minced

Minced fresh ginger – 2 tsp.

Fresh pea pods – 4 cups, trimmed

Homemade soy sauce – 3 Tbsp.

Cooked brown rice – 4 cups

Method

1.   Heat the oil in a pan.

2.   Add the garlic, scallions, and ginger.

3.	Stir-fry for 30 seconds.

4.	Add the sliced beef and stir-fry for 5 minutes, or until beef has browned.

5.	Add pea pods and soy sauce and stir-fry for 3 minutes.

6.	Remove from heat.

7.	Serve with rice.

Homemade soy sauce

Molasses – ¼ cup

Unflavored rice wine vinegar – 3 Tbsp.

Water – 1 Tbsp.

Sodium-free beef bouillon granules – 1 tsp.

Freshly ground black pepper - ½ tsp.

Method

1.	Mix everything in a saucepan and heat on low for 1 minute.

2.	Serve.

Nutritional Facts Per Serving

Calories: 466

Fat: 11g

Carb: 64g

Protein: 27g

Sodium 71mg

Whole-Grain Rotini with Ground Pork

Prep time: 10 minutes

Cook time: 25 minutes

Servings: 6

Ingredients

Whole-grain rotini - 1 (13-ounce) package

Lean ground pork – 1 pound

Red onion – 1, chopped

Garlic – 3 cloves, minced

Bell pepper – 1, chopped

Pumpkin puree – 1 cup Ground sage – 2 tsp.

Ground rosemary – 1 tsp.

Ground black pepper to taste

Method

1.   Cook the pasta (follow the package insturctions). Omit salt, drain and set aside.

2. Heat a pan over medium heat. Add onion, garlic, and ground pork and sauté for 2 minutes.

3. Add bell pepper and sauté for 5 minutes.

4. Remove from heat. Add pasta to the pan along with remaining ingredients.

5. Mix and serve.

Nutritional Facts Per Serving

Calories: 331

Fat: 7g

Carb: 45g

Protein: 23g

Sodium 48mg

Roasted Pork Loin with Herbs

Prep time: 20 minutes

Cook time: 1 hour

Servings: 4

Ingredients

Boneless pork loin roast – 2 lbs.

Garlic – 3 cloves, minced Dried rosemary – 1 Tbsp.

Dried thyme – 1 tsp.

Dried basil – 1 tsp.

Salt – ¼ tsp.

Olive oil – ¼ cup

White wine – ½ cup Pepper to taste

Method

1.   Preheat the oven to 350F.

2.   Crush the garlic with thyme, rosemary, basil, salt, and pepper, making a paste. Set aside.

3.   Use a knife to pierce meat several times.

4.	Press the garlic paste into the slits.

5.	Rub the meat with the rest of the garlic mixture and olive oil.

6.	Place pork loin into the oven, turning and basting with pan liquids, until the pork reaches 145F, about 1 hour. Remove the pork from the oven.

7.	Place the pan over heat and add white wine, stirring the brown bits on the bottom.

8.	Top roast with sauce.

9.	Serve.

Nutritional Facts Per Serving

Calories: 464

Fat: 20.7g

Carb: 2.4g

Protein: 59.6g

Sodium 279mg

Garlic Lime Pork Chops

Prep time: 20 minutes

Cook time: 10 minutes

Servings: 4

Ingredients

Lean boneless pork chops – 4 (6-oz. each)

Garlic – 4 cloves, crushed Cumin – ½ tsp.

Chili powder - ½ tsp.

Paprika - ½ tsp.

Juice of ½ lime Lime zest – 1 tsp.

Kosher salt - ¼ tsp.

Fresh pepper to taste

Method

1.   In a bowl, season pork with cumin, chili powder, paprika, garlic salt, and pepper. Add lime juice and zest.

2.   Marinate the pork for 20 minutes.

3.   Line a broiler pan with foil.

4.   Place the pork chops on the broiler pan and broil for 5 minutes on each side or until browned.

5.   Serve.

Nutritional Facts Per Serving

Calories: 233

Fat: 13.2g

Carb: 4.3g

Protein: 25.5g

Sodium 592mg

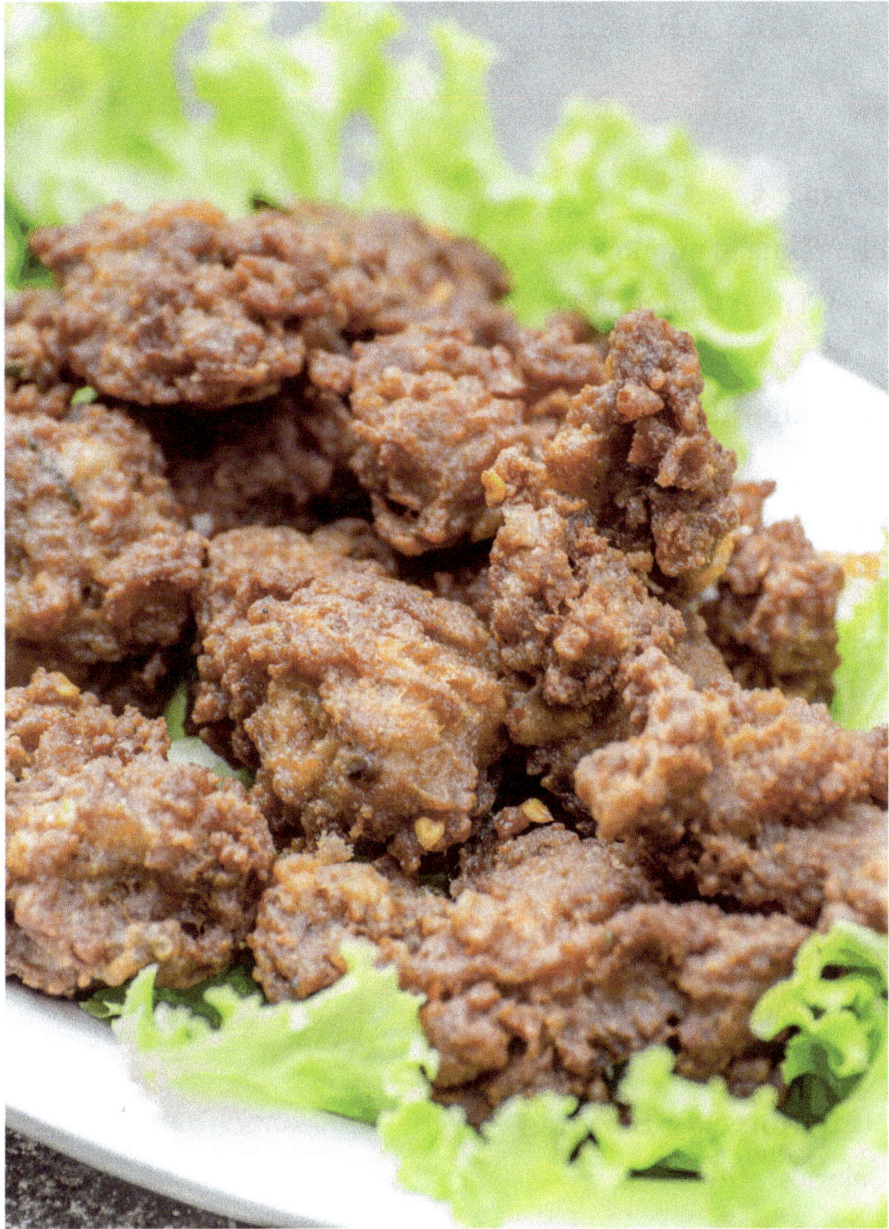

The Most Elegant Parsley Soufflé Ever

Serving: 5

Prep Time: 5 minutes

Cook Time: 6 minutes

Ingredients:

2 whole eggs

1 fresh red chili pepper, chopped

2 tablespoons coconut cream

1 tablespoon fresh parsley, chopped Sunflower seeds to taste

How To:

1. Pre-heat your oven to 390 degrees F.

2.   Almond butter 2 soufflé dishes.

3.   Add the ingredients to a blender and mix well.

4.   Divide batter into soufflé dishes and bake for 6 minutes.

5.   Serve and enjoy!

Nutrition (Per Serving)

Calories: 108

Fat: 9g

Carbohydrates: 9g

Protein: 6g

Fennel and Almond Bites

Serving: 12

Prep Time: 10 minutes

Cooking Time: None

Freeze Time: 3 hours

Ingredients:

1 teaspoon vanilla extract

¼ cup almond milk

¼ cup cocoa powder

½ cup almond oil

A pinch of sunflower seeds

1 teaspoon fennel seeds

How To:

1.   Take a bowl and mix the almond oil and almond milk.

2.   Beat until smooth and glossy using electric beater.

3.   Mix in the rest of the ingredients.

4.   Take a piping bag and pour into a parchment paper lined baking sheet.

5.   Freeze for 3 hours and store in the fridge.

Nutrition (Per Serving)

Total Carbs: 1g

Fiber: 1g

Protein: 1g

Fat: 20g

Feisty Coconut Fudge

Serving: 12

Prep Time: 20 minutes

Cooking Time: None

Freeze Time: 2 hours

Ingredients:

¼ cup coconut, shredded

2 cups coconut oil

½ cup coconut cream

¼ cup almonds, chopped

1 teaspoon almond extract

A pinch of sunflower seeds

Stevia to taste

How To:

1.   Take a large bowl and pour coconut cream and coconut oil into it.

2.   Whisk using an electric beater.

3.   Whisk until the mixture becomes smooth and glossy.

4.   Add cocoa powder slowly and mix well.

5.   Add in the rest of the ingredients.

6.   Pour into a bread pan lined with parchment paper.

7.   Freeze until set.

8.   Cut them into squares and serve.

Nutrition (Per Serving)

Total Carbs: 1g

Fiber: 1g

Protein: 0g

Fat: 20g

No Bake Cheesecake

Serving: 10

Prep Time: 120 minutes

Cook Time: Nil

Ingredients:

For Crust

2 tablespoons ground flaxseeds

2 tablespoons desiccated coconut

1 teaspoon cinnamon

For Filling

4 ounces vegan cream cheese

1 cup cashews, soaked

½ cup frozen blueberries

2 tablespoons coconut oil

1 tablespoon lemon juice

1 teaspoon vanilla extract Liquid stevia

How To:

1.   Take a container and mix in the crust ingredients, mix well.

2.   Flatten the mixture at the bottom to prepare the crust of your cheesecake.

3.   Take a blender/ food processor and add the filling ingredients, blend until smooth.

4.   Gently pour the batter on top of your crust and chill for 2 hours.

5.   Serve and enjoy!

Nutrition (Per Serving)

Calories: 182

Fat: 16g

Carbohydrates: 4g

Protein: 3g

Easy Chia Seed Pumpkin Pudding

Serving: 4

Prep Time: 10-15 minutes/ overnight chill time

Cook Time: Nil

Ingredients:

1 cup maple syrup

2 teaspoons pumpkin spice

1 cup pumpkin puree

1 ¼ cup almond milk

½ cup chia seeds

How To:

1.   Add all of the ingredients to a bowl and gently stir.

2.   Let it refrigerate overnight or at least 15 minutes.

3.   Top with your desired ingredients, such as blueberries, almonds, etc.

4.   Serve and enjoy!

Nutrition (Per Serving)

Calories: 230

Fat: 10g

Carbohydrates:22g

Protein:11g

Lovely Blueberry Pudding

Serving: 4

Prep Time: 20 minutes

Cook Time: Nil

Ingredients:

2 cups frozen blueberries

2 teaspoons lime zest, grated freshly

20 drops liquid stevia

2 small avocados, peeled, pitted and chopped ½ teaspoon fresh ginger, grated freshly

4 tablespoons fresh lime juice

10 tablespoons water

How To:

1.   Add all of the listed ingredients to a blender (except blueberries) and pulse the mixture well.

2.   Transfer the mix into small serving bowls and chill the bowls.

3.   Serve with a topping of blueberries.

4.   Enjoy!

Nutrition (Per Serving)

Calories: 166

Fat: 13g

Carbohydrates: 13g

Protein: 1.7g

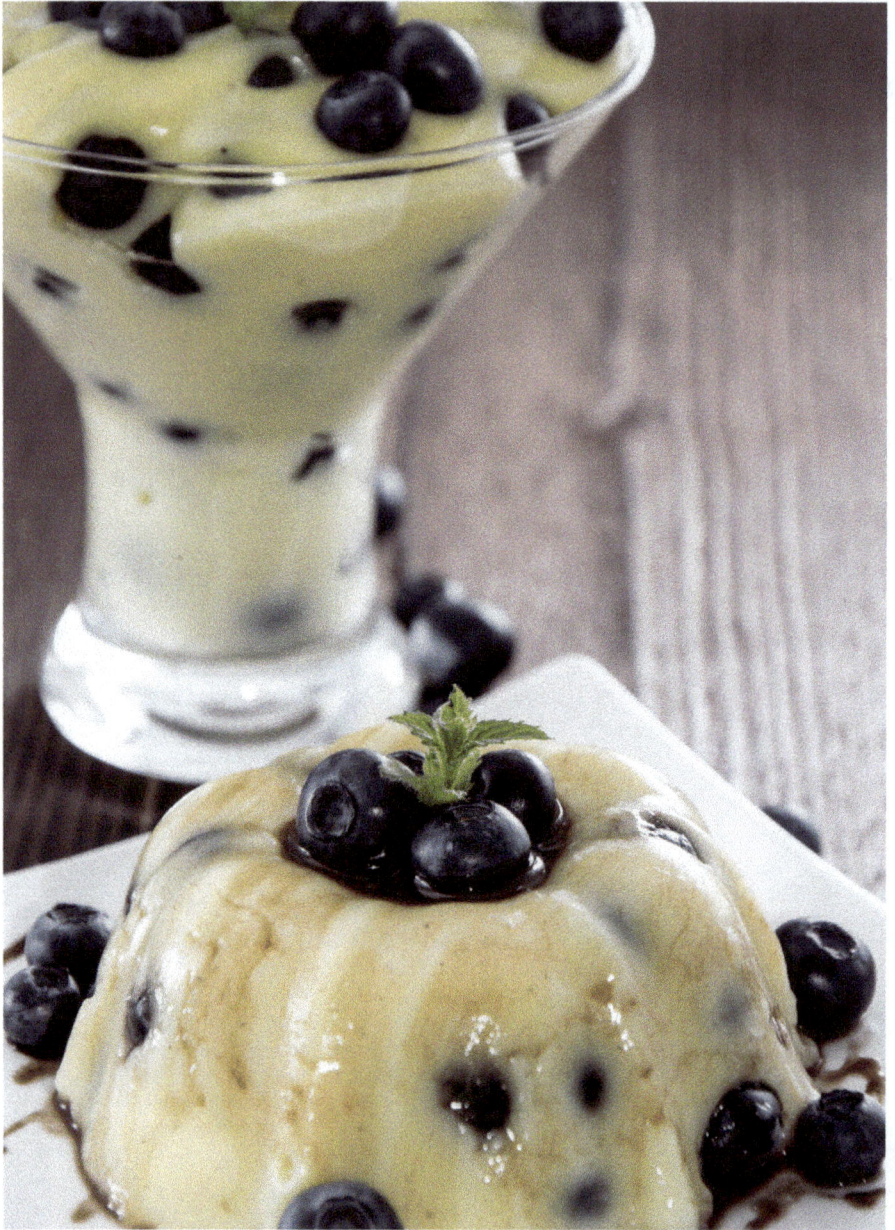

Decisive Lime and Strawberry Popsicle

Serving: 4

Prep Time: 2 hours

Cook Time: Nil

Ingredients:

1 tablespoon lime juice, fresh

¼ cup strawberries, hulled and sliced

¼ cup coconut almond milk, unsweetened and full fat 2 teaspoons natural sweetener

How To:

1.   Blend the listed ingredients in a blender until smooth.

2.   Pour mix into popsicle molds and let them chill for 2 hours.

3.   Serve and enjoy!

Nutrition (Per Serving)

Calories: 166

Fat: 17g

Carbohydrates: 3g

Protein: 1g

Authentic Ginger and Berry Smoothie

Serving: 2

Prep Time: 5 minutes

Cook Time: Nil

Ingredients:

2 cups blackberries

2 cups unsweetened almond milk

1 -2 packs of stevia

1 piece of 1-inch fresh ginger, peeled and roughly chopped

2 cups crushed ice

How To:

1.   Add the listed ingredients to a blender and blend the whole mixture until smooth.

2.   Serve chilled and enjoy!

Nutrition (Per Serving)

Calories: 200

Fat: 10g

Carbohydrates: 14g

Protein 2g

A Glassful of Kale and Spinach

Serving: 2

Prep Time: 5 minutes

Ingredients:

Handful of kale

Handful of spinach

2 broccoli heads

1 tomato

Handful of lettuce

1 avocado, cubed

1 cucumber, cubed

Juice of ½ lemon

Pineapple juice as needed

How To:

1.   Add all the listed ingredients to your blender.

2.   Blend until smooth.

3.   Add a few ice cubes and serve the smoothie.

4.   Enjoy!

Nutrition (Per Serving)

Calories: 200

Fat: 10g

Carbohydrates: 14g

Protein 2g

Green Tea, Turmeric, and Mango Smoothie

Serving: 2

Prep Time: 5 minutes

Ingredients:

2 cups mango, cubed

2 teaspoons turmeric powder

2 tablespoons Green Tea powder

2 cups almond milk

2 tablespoons honey

1 cup crushed ice

How To:

1.   Add the listed ingredients to a blender and blend the whole mixture until smooth.

2.   Serve chilled and enjoy!

Nutrition (Per Serving)

Calories: 200

Fat: 10g

Carbohydrates: 14g

Protein 2g

The Great Anti-Oxidant Glass

Serving: 2

Prep Time: 5 minutes

Ingredients:

1 whole ripe avocado

4 cups organic baby spinach leaves

1 cup filtered water

Juice of 1 lemon

1 English cucumber, chopped

3 stems fresh parsley

5 stems fresh mint

1-inch piece fresh ginger

2 large ice cubes

How To:

1.   Add all the listed ingredients to your blender.

2.   Blend until smooth.

3.   Add a few ice cubes and serve the smoothie.

4.   Enjoy!

Nutrition (Per Serving)

Calories: 200

Fat: 10g

Carbohydrates: 14g

Protein 2g

Fresh Minty Smoothie

Serving: 1

Prep Time: 10 minutes

Ingredients:

1 stalk celery

2 cups water

2 ounces almonds

1 packet stevia

1 cup spinach

2 mint leaves

How To:

1.   Add listed ingredients to blender.

2.   Blend until you have a smooth and creamy texture.

3.   Serve chilled and enjoy!

Nutrition (Per Serving)

Calories: 417

Fat: 43g

Carbohydrates: 10g

Protein: 5.5g

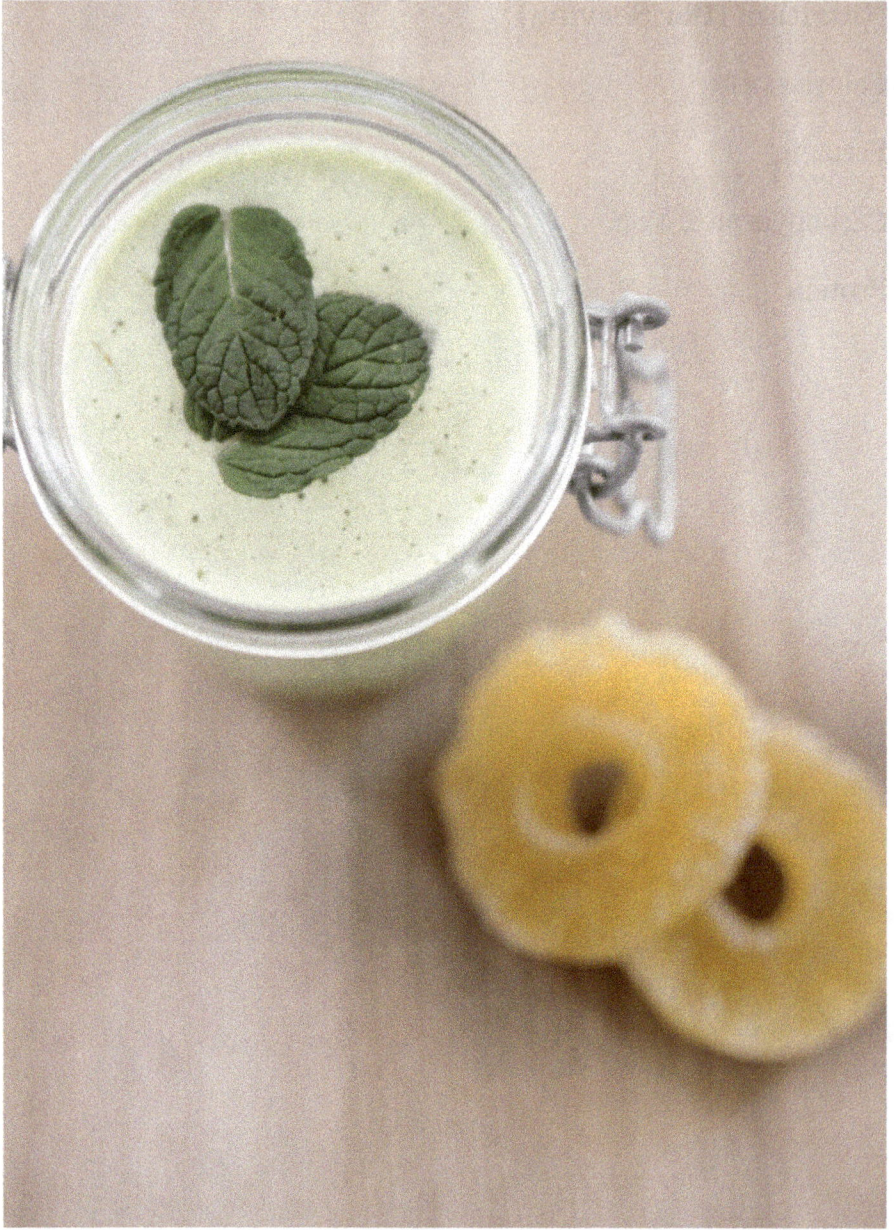

Apple Slices

Serving: 4

Prep Time: 10 minutes

Cook Time: 10 minutes

Ingredients:

1 cup of coconut oil

¼ cup date paste

2 tablespoons ground cinnamon

4 granny smith apples, peeled and sliced, cored

How To:

1.   Take a large sized skillet and place it over medium heat.

2.   Add oil and allow the oil to heat up.

3.   Stir in cinnamon and date paste into the oil.

4.   Add cut up apples and cook for 5-8 minutes until crispy.

5.   Serve and enjoy!

Nutrition (Per Serving)

Calories: 368

Fat: 23g

Carbohydrates: 44g

Protein: 1g

Elegant Cashew Sauce

Serving: 4

Prep Time: 5 minutes

Cook Time: Nil

Ingredients:

3 ounces cashew nuts

¼ cup water

½ cup olive oil

1 tablespoons lemon juice

½ teaspoon onion powder

½ teaspoon sunflower seeds

1 pinch cayenne pepper

How To:

Add nuts to your blender and process.

Add other ingredients (except oil) and process until smooth.

Add a little bit of oil and puree.

Serve as needed!

Nutrition (Per Serving)

Calories: 361

Fat: 37g

Carbohydrates: 6g

Protein: 3g

Lovely Japanese Cabbage Dish

Serving: 6

Prep Time: 25 minutes

Cook Time: Nil

Ingredients:

3 tablespoons sesame oil

3 tablespoons rice vinegar

1 garlic clove, minced

1 teaspoon fresh ginger root, grated

1 teaspoon sunflower seeds

1 teaspoon pepper

½ large head cabbage, cored and shredded 1 bunch green onions, thinly sliced 1 cup almond slivers

¼ cup toasted sesame seeds

How To:

1.   Add all listed ingredients to a large bowl, making sure to add the wet ingredients first, followed by the dried ingredients.

2. Toss well to ensure that the cabbages are coated well.

3. Let it chill and enjoy!

Nutrition (Per Serving)

Calories: 126

Fat: 10g

Carbohydrates: 9g

Protein: 4g

Almond Buttery Green Cabbage

Serving: 4

Prep Time: 10 minutes

Cook Time: 15 minutes

Ingredients:

1 ½ pounds shredded green cabbage

3 ounces almond butter

Sunflower seeds and pepper to taste

1 dollop, whipped cream

How To:

1.   Take a large skillet and place it over medium heat.

2.   Add almond butter and melt.

3.   Stir in cabbage and sauté for 15 minutes.

4.   Season accordingly.

5.   Serve with a dollop of cream.

6.   Enjoy!

Nutrition (Per Serving)

Calories: 199

Fat: 17g

Carbohydrates: 10g

Protein: 3g

Chia Porridge

Serving: 2

Prep Time: 10 minutes

Cook Time: 5-10 minutes

Ingredients:

1 tablespoon chia seeds

1 tablespoon ground flaxseed

1/3 cup coconut cream

½ cup water

1 teaspoon vanilla extract

1 tablespoon almond butter

How To:

1.   Add chia seeds, coconut milk, flaxseed, water and vanilla to a little pot.

2.   Stir and let it sit for five minutes.

3.   Add almond butter and place pot over low heat.

4.   Keep stirring as almond butter melts.

5. Once the porridge is hot/not boiling, pour into bowl.

6. Enjoy!

7. Add a couple of berries or a touch of cream for extra flavor.

Nutrition (Per Serving)

Calories: 410

Fat: 38g

Carbohydrates: 10g

Protein: 6g

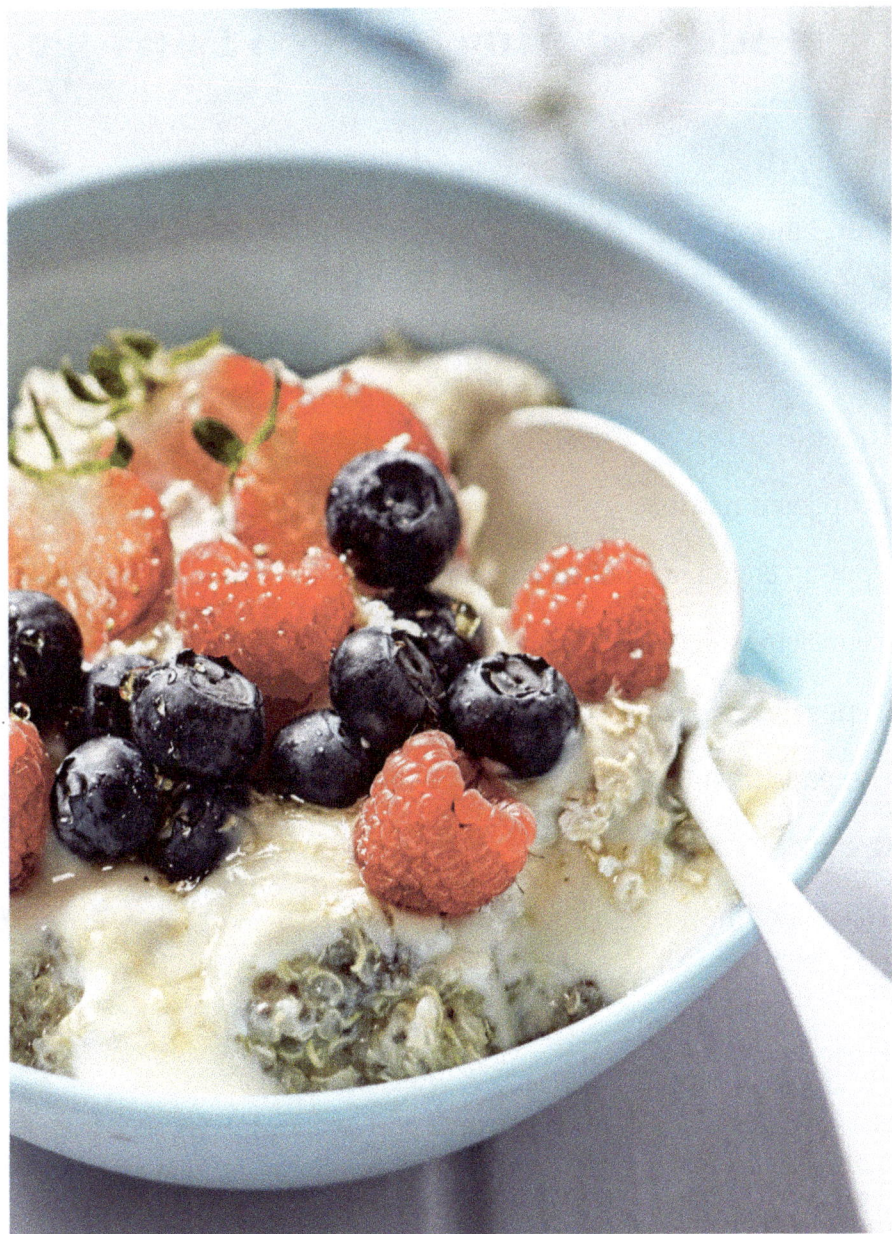

Mouthwatering Chicken Porridge

Serving: 4

Prep Time: 1 hour

Cook Time: 10-20 minutes

Ingredients:

1 cup jasmine rice

1 pound steamed/cooked chicken legs

5 cups chicken broth

4 cups water

1 ½ cups fresh ginger

Green onions

Toasted cashew nuts

How To:

1.   Place the rice in your fridge and permit it to relax 1 hour before cooking.

2.   Take the rice out and add it to your Instant Pot.

3.   Pour in chicken stock and water.

4.   Lock the lid and cook on PORRIDGE mode, using the default settings and parameters.

5.   Release the pressure naturally over 10 minutes.

6.   Open the lid.

7.   Remove the meat from the chicken legs and add the meat to your soup.

8.   Stir overflow Sauté mode.

9.   Season with a touch of flavored vinegar and luxuriate in with a garnish of nuts and onion.

Nutrition (Per Serving)

Calories: 206

Fat: 8g

Carbohydrates: 8g

Protein: 23g

Simple Blueberry Oatmeal

Serving: 4

Prep Time: 10 minutes

Cooking Time: 8 hours

Ingredients:

1 cup blueberries

1 cup steel-cut oats1 cup coconut milk

2 tablespoons agave nectar

½ teaspoon vanilla extract Coconut flakes, garnish

How To:

1.   Grease Slow Cooker with cooking spray.

2.   Add oats, milk, nectar, blueberries, and vanilla.

3.   Toss well.

4.   Place lid and cook on LOW for 8 hours.

5.   Divide between serving bowls and serve.

6.   Enjoy!

Nutrition (Per Serving)

Calories: 202

Fat: 6g

Carbohydrates: 12g

Protein: 6g

The Decisive Apple "Porridge"

Serving: 2

Prep Time: 10 minutes

Cook Time: 5 minutes

Ingredients:

1 large apple, peeled, cored and grated

1 cup unsweetened almond milk

1 ½ tablespoons sunflower seeds

1/8 cup fresh blueberries

¼ teaspoon fresh vanilla bean extract

How To:

1.   Take an outsized pan and add sunflower seeds, vanilla, almond milk, apples, and stir.

2.   Place over medium-low heat.

3.   Cook for five minutes, ensuring to stay the mixture stirring.

4.   Transfer to a serving bowl.

5.   Serve and enjoy!

Nutrition (Per Serving)

Calories: 123

Fat: 1.3g

Carbohydrates:23g

Protein: 4g

The Unique Smoothie Bowl

Serving: 2

Prep Time: 10 minutes

Cook Time: Nil

Ingredients:

2 cups baby spinach leaves

1 cup coconut almond milk

¼ cup low fat cream

2 tablespoons flaxseed oil

2 tablespoons chia seeds

2 tablespoons walnuts, roughly chopped A handful of fresh berries

How To:

1.   Add spinach leaves, coconut almond milk, cream and linseed oil to a blender.

2.   Blitz until smooth.

3.   Pour smoothie into serving bowls.

4.   Sprinkle chia seeds, berries, walnuts on top.

5.   Serve and enjoy!

Nutrition (Per Serving)

Calories: 380

Fat: 36g

Carbohydrates: 12g

Protein: 5g

Cinnamon and Coconut Porridge

Serving: 4

Prep Time: 5 minutes

Cook Time:5 minutes

Ingredients:

2 cups water

1 cup coconut cream

½ cup unsweetened dried coconut, shredded 2 tablespoons flaxseed meal 1 tablespoon almond butter

1 ½ teaspoons stevia

1 teaspoon cinnamon

Toppings as blueberries

How To:

1.   Add the listed ingredients to a little pot, mix well.

2.   Transfer pot to stove and place over medium-low heat.

3.   bring back mix to a slow boil.

4.   Stir well and take away from the warmth.

5.   Divide the combination into equal servings and allow them to sit for 10 minutes.

6.   Top together with your desired toppings and enjoy!

Nutrition (Per Serving)

Calories: 171

Fat: 16g

Carbohydrates: 6g

Protein: 2g

Morning Porridge

Serving: 2

Prep Time: 15 minutes

Cook Time: Nil

Ingredients:

2 tablespoons coconut flour

2 tablespoons vanilla protein powder

3 tablespoons Golden Flaxseed meal

1 ½ cups almond milk, unsweetened Powdered erythritol

How To:

1.   Take a bowl and blend in flaxseed meal, protein powder, coconut flour and blend well.

2.   Add mix to the saucepan (place over medium heat).

3.   Add almond milk and stir, let the mixture thicken.

4.   Add your required amount of sweetener and serve.

5.   Enjoy!

Nutrition (Per Serving)

Calories: 259

Fat: 13g

Carbohydrates: 5g

Protein: 16g

Tantalizing Cauliflower and Dill Mash

Serving: 6

Prep Time: 10 minutes

Cooking Time: 6 hours

Ingredients:

1 cauliflower head, florets separated

1/3 cup dill, chopped

6 garlic cloves

2 tablespoons olive oil

Pinch of black pepper

How To:

1.	Add cauliflower to Slow Cooker.

2.	Add dill, garlic and water to hide them. 3. Place lid and cook on HIGH for five hours.

3.	Drain the flowers.

4.	Season with pepper and add oil, mash using potato masher.

5.   Whisk and serve.

6.   Enjoy!

Nutrition (Per Serving)

Calories: 207

Fat: 4g

Carbohydrates: 14g

Protein: 3g

Secret Asian Green Beans

Serving: 10

Prep Time: 10 minutes

Cooking Time: 2 hours

Ingredients:

16 cups green beans, halved

3 tablespoons olive oil

¼ cup tomato sauce, salt-free

½ cup coconut sugar

¾ teaspoon low sodium soy sauce

Pinch of pepper

How To:

1.   Add green beans, coconut sugar, pepper spaghetti sauce , soy sauce, oil to your Slow Cooker.

2.   Stir well.

3.   Place lid and cook on LOW for 3 hours.

4.   Divide between serving platters and serve.

5.   Enjoy!

Nutrition (Per Serving)

Calories: 200

Fat: 4g

Carbohydrates: 12g

Protein: 3g

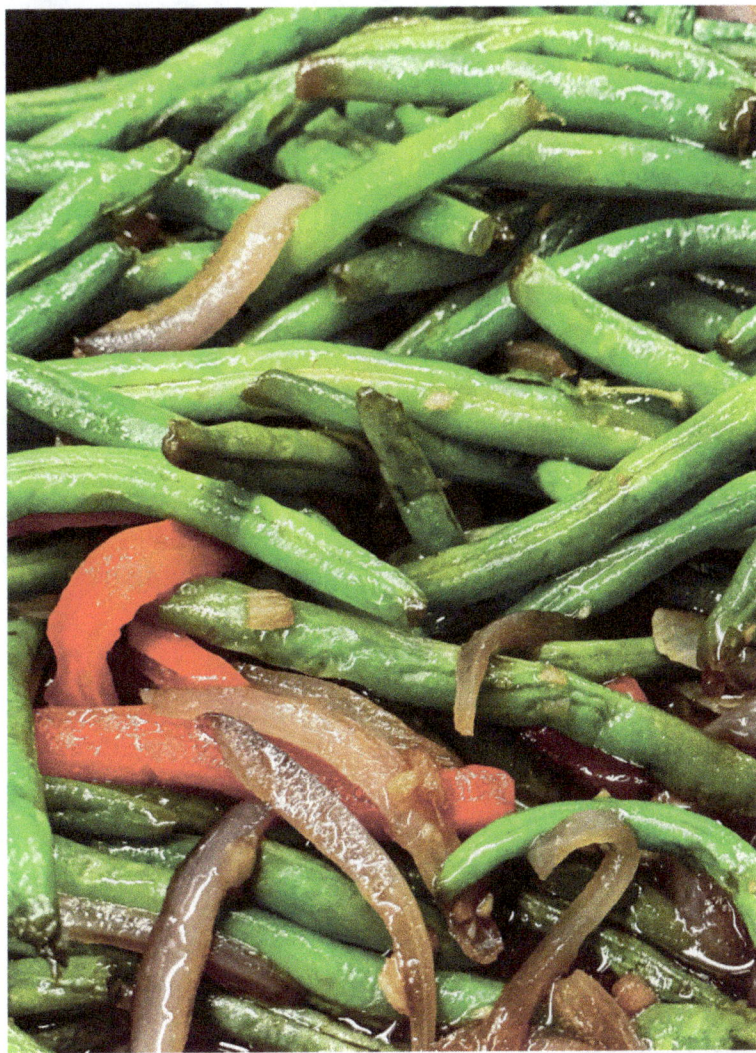

Excellent Acorn Mix

Serving: 10

Prep Time: 10 minutes

Cooking Time: 7 hours

Ingredients:

2 acorn squash, peeled and cut into wedges

16 ounces cranberry sauce, unsweetened

¼ teaspoon cinnamon powder Pepper to taste

How To:

1. Add acorn wedges to your Slow Cooker.

2. Add condiment, cinnamon, raisins and pepper.

3. Stir.

4. Place lid and cook on LOW for 7 hours.

5. Serve and enjoy!

Nutrition (Per Serving)

Calories: 200

Fat: 3g

Carbohydrates: 15g

Protein: 2g

Crunchy Almond Chocolate Bars

Serving: 12

Prep Time: 10 minutes

Cooking Time: 2 hours 30 minutes

Ingredients:

1 egg white

¼ cup coconut oil, melted

1 cup coconut sugar

½ teaspoon vanilla extract

1 teaspoon baking powder

1 ½ cups almond meal

½ cup dark chocolate chips

How To:

1.   Take a bowl and add sugar, oil, vanilla, egg white, almond flour, leaven and blend it well.

2.   Fold in chocolate chips and stir.

3.   Line Slow Cooker with parchment paper.

4.   Grease.

5.   Add the cookie mix and continue bottom.

6.   Place lid and cook on LOW for two hours half-hour .

7.   Take cooking utensil out and let it cool.

8. Cut in bars and enjoy!

Nutrition (Per Serving)

Calories: 200

Fat: 2g

Carbohydrates: 13g

Protein: 6g

Lettuce and Chicken Platter

Serving: 6

Prep Time: 10 minutes

Cook Time: nil

Ingredients:

2 cups chicken, cooked and coarsely chopped ½ head ice berg lettuce, sliced and chopped 1 celery rib, chopped

1 medium apple, cut

½ red bell pepper, deseeded and chopped 6-7 green olives, pitted and halved 1 red onion, chopped

For dressing

1 tablespoon raw honey

2 tablespoons lemon juice

Salt and pepper to taste

How To:

1.   Cut the vegetables and transfer them to your Salad Bowl.

2.   Add olives.

3.   Chop the cooked chicken and transfer to your Salad bowl.

4.   Prepare dressing by mixing the ingredients listed under Dressing.

5.   Pour the dressing into the Salad bowl.

6.   Toss and enjoy!

Nutrition (Per Serving)

Calories: 296

Fat: 21g

Carbohydrates: 9g

Protein: 18g

Chipotle Lettuce Chicken

Serving: 6

Prep Time: 10 minutes

Cook Time: 25 minutes

Ingredients:

1-pound chicken breast, cut into strips

Splash of olive oil

1 red onion, finely sliced

14 ounces tomatoes

1 teaspoon chipotle, chopped

½ teaspoon cumin

Lettuce as needed

Fresh coriander leaves

Jalapeno chilies, sliced

Fresh tomato slices for garnish

Lime wedges

How To:

1. Take a non-stick frypan and place it over medium heat.

2. Add oil and warmth it up.

3. Add chicken and cook until brown.

4. Keep the chicken on the side.

5. Add tomatoes, sugar, chipotle, cumin to an equivalent pan and simmer for 25 minutes until you've got a pleasant sauce.

6. Add chicken into the sauce and cook for five minutes.

7. Transfer the combination to a different place.

8. Use lettuce wraps to require some of the mixture and serve with a squeeze of lemon.

9. Enjoy!

Nutrition (Per Serving)

Calories: 332

Fat: 15g

Carbohydrates: 13g

Protein: 34g

Balsamic Chicken and Vegetables

Serving: 2

Prep Time: 15 minutes

Cook Time: 25 minutes

Ingredients:

4 chicken thigh, boneless and skinless

5 stalks of asparagus, halved

1 pepper, cut in chunks

1/2 red onion, diced

½ cup carrots, sliced

1 garlic clove, minced

2-ounces mushrooms, diced

¼ cup balsamic vinegar

1 tablespoon olive oil

½ teaspoon stevia

½ tablespoon oregano

Sunflower seeds and pepper as needed

How To:

1. Pre-heat your oven to 425 degrees F.

2.   Take a bowl and add all of the vegetables and blend.

3.   Add spices and oil and blend.

4.   Dip the chicken pieces into spice mix and coat them well.

5.   Place the veggies and chicken onto a pan during a single layer.

6.   Cook for 25 minutes.

7.   Serve and enjoy!

Nutrition (Per Serving)

Calories: 401

Fat: 17g

Net Carbohydrates: 11g

Protein: 48g

Cream Dredged Corn Platter

Serving: 3

Prep Time: 10 minutes

Cook Time: 4 hours

Ingredients:

3 cups corn

2 ounces cream cheese, cubed

2 tablespoons milk

2 tablespoons whipping cream

2 tablespoons butter, melted

Salt and pepper as needed

1 tablespoon green onion, chopped

How To:

1.   Add corn, cheese, milk, light whipping cream, butter, salt and pepper to your Slow Cooker.

2.   provides it a pleasant toss to combine everything well.

3.   Place lid and cook on LOW for 4 hours.

4.   Divide the combination amongst serving platters.

5.   Serve and enjoy!

Nutrition (Per Serving)

Calories: 261

Fat: 11g

Carbohydrates: 17g

Protein: 6g

Exuberant Sweet Potatoes

Serving: 4

Prep Time: 5 minutes

Cook Time: 7-8 hours

Ingredients:

6 sweet potatoes, washed and dried

How To:

1.   Loosely botch 7-8 pieces of aluminium foil within the bottom of your Slow Cooker, covering about half the area.

2.   Prick each potato 6-8 times employing a fork.

3.   Wrap each potato with foil and seal them.

4.   Place wrapped potatoes within the cooker on top of the foil bed.

5.   Place lid and cook on LOW for 7-8 hours.

6.   Use tongs to get rid of the potatoes and unwrap them.

7.   Serve and enjoy!

Nutrition (Per Serving)

Calories: 129

Fat: 0g

Carbohydrates: 30g

Protein: 2g

Leek and Cauliflower Soup

Serving: 6

Prep Time: 10 minutes

Cook Time: 40 minutes

Ingredients:

3 cups cauliflower, riced

1 bay leaf

1 teaspoon herbs de Provence

2 garlic cloves, peeled and diced

½ cup coconut milk

2 ½ cups vegetable stock

1 tablespoon coconut oil

½ teaspoon cracked pepper

1 leek, chopped

How To:

1.   Take a pot, heat oil into it.

2.   Sauté the leeks in the oil for 5 minutes.

3.   Add the garlic and then stir-cook for another minute.

4.   Add all the remaining ingredients and mix them well.

5.   Cook for 30 minutes.

6.   Stir occasionally.

7.   Blend the soup until smooth by using an immersion blender.

8.   Serve hot and enjoy!

Nutrition (Per Serving)

Calories: 90

Fat: 7g

Carbohydrates: 4g

Protein: 2g

Dreamy Zucchini Bowl

Serving: 4

Prep Time: 10 minutes

Cook Time: 20 minutes

Ingredients:

1 onion, chopped

3 zucchini, cut into medium chunks

2 tablespoons coconut almond milk

2 garlic cloves, minced

4 cups vegetable stock

2 tablespoons coconut oil

Pinch of sunflower seeds

Black pepper to taste

How To:

1.   Take a pot and place it over medium heat.

2.   Add oil and let it heat up.

3.   Add zucchini, garlic, onion and stir.

4.   Cook for 5 minutes.

5.   Add stock, sunflower seeds, pepper and stir.

6.   Bring to a boil and reduce heat.

7.   Simmer for 20 minutes.

8.   Remove from heat and add coconut almond milk.

9.   Use an immersion blender until smooth.

10.   Ladle into soup bowls and serve.

11.   Enjoy!

Nutrition (Per Serving)

Calories: 160

Fat: 2g

Carbohydrates: 4g

Protein: 7g

Cold Crab and Watermelon Soup

Serving: 4

Prep Time: 10 minutes + chill time

Cook Time: nil

Ingredients:

¼ cup basil, chopped

2 pounds tomatoes

5 cups watermelon, cubed

¼ cup wine vinegar

2 garlic cloves, minced

1 zucchini, chopped

Pepper to taste

1 cup crabmeat

How To:

1.   Take your blender and add tomatoes, basil, vinegar, 4 cups watermelon, garlic, 1/3 cup oil, pepper and pulse well.

2.   Transfer to fridge and chill for 1 hour.

3.   Divide into bowls and add zucchini, crab and remaining watermelon.

4.   Serve and enjoy!

Nutrition (Per Serving)

Calories: 121

Fat: 3g

Carbohydrates: 4g

Protein: 8g

Paleo Lemon and Garlic Soup

Serving: 4

Prep Time: 10 minutes

Cook Time: 10 minutes

Ingredients:

6 cups shellfish stock

1 tablespoon garlic, minced

1 tablespoon coconut oil, melted

2 whole eggs

½ cup lemon juice

Pinch of salt

White pepper to taste

1 tablespoon arrowroot powder

Finely chopped cilantro for serving

How To:

1.   Heat up a pot with oil over medium high heat.

2.   Add garlic, stir cook for 2 minutes.

3.   Add stock (reserve ½ cup for later use).

4.   Stir and bring mix to a simmer.

5.   Take a bowl and add eggs, sea salt, pepper, reserved stock, lemon juice and arrowroot.

6.   Whisk well.

7.   Pour in to the soup and cook for a few minutes.

8.   Ladle soup into bowls and serve with chopped cilantro.

9.   Enjoy!

Nutrition (Per Serving)

Calories: 135

Fat: 3g

Carbohydrates: 12g

Protein: 8

Brussels Soup

Serving: 4

Prep Time: 10 minutes

Cook Time: 20 minutes

Ingredients:

2 tablespoons olive oil

1 yellow onion, chopped

2 pounds Brussels sprouts, trimmed and halved

4 cups chicken stock

¼ cup coconut cream

How To:

1.   Take a pot and place it over medium heat.

2.   Add oil and let it heat up.

3.   Add onion and stir-cook for 3 minutes.

4.   Add Brussels sprouts and stir, cook for 2 minutes.

5.   Add stock and black pepper, stir and bring to a simmer.

6.   Cook for 20 minutes more.

7.   Use an immersion blender to make the soup creamy.

8.   Add coconut cream and stir well.

9.   Ladle into soup bowls and serve.

10.   Enjoy!

Nutrition (Per Serving)

Calories: 200

Fat: 11g

Carbohydrates: 6g

Protein: 11g

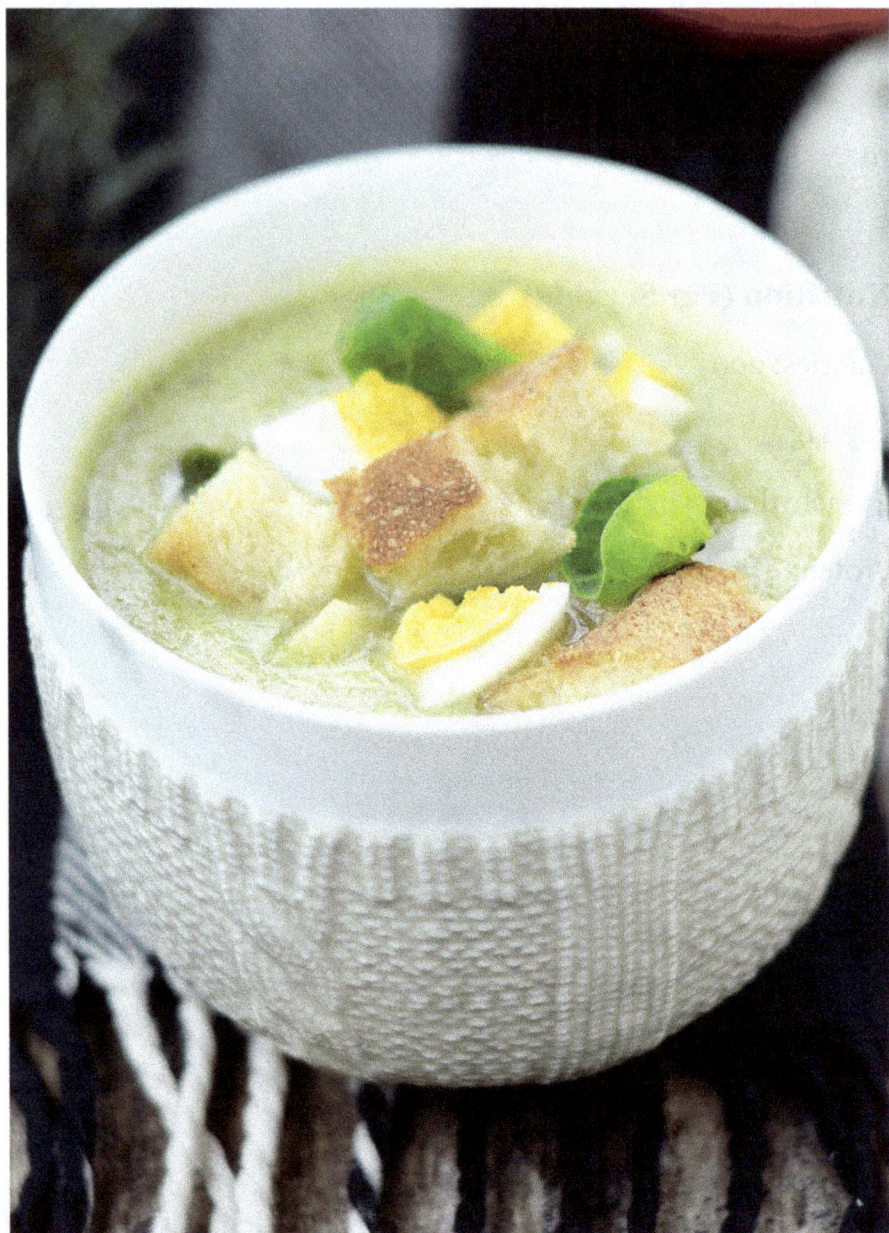

Spring Soup and Poached Egg

Serving: 4

Prep Time: 5 minutes

Cook Time: 15 minutes

Ingredients:

2 whole eggs

32 ounces chicken broth

1 head romaine lettuce, chopped

How To:

1.   Bring the chicken broth to a boil.

2.   Reduce the heat and poach the 2 eggs in the broth for 5 minutes.

3.   Take two bowls and transfer the eggs into a separate bowl.

4.   Add chopped romaine lettuce into the broth and cook for a few minutes.

5.   Serve the broth with lettuce into the bowls.

6.   Enjoy!

Nutrition (Per Serving)

Calories: 150

Fat: 5g

Carbohydrates: 6g

Protein: 16g

Lobster Bisque

Serving: 4

Prep Time: 10 minutes

Cook Time: 15 minutes

Ingredients:

¾ pound lobster, cooked and lobster

4 cups chicken broth

2 garlic cloves, chopped

¼ teaspoon pepper

½ teaspoon paprika

1 yellow onion, chopped

½ teaspoon salt

14 ½ ounces tomatoes, diced

1 tablespoon coconut oil

1 cup low fat cream

How To:

1.   Take a stockpot and add the coconut oil over medium heat.

2.   Then sauté the garlic and onion for 3 to 5 minutes.

3.   Add diced tomatoes, spices and chicken broth and bring to a boil.

4.   Reduce to a simmer, then simmer for about 10 minutes.

5.   Add the warmed heavy cream to the soup.

6.   Blend the soup till creamy by using an immersion blender.

7.   Stir in cooked lobster.

8.   Serve and enjoy!

Nutrition (Per Serving)

Calories: 180

Fat: 11g

Carbohydrates: 6g

Protein: 16g

Tomato Bisque

Serving: 4

Prep Time: 10 minutes

Cook Time: 40 minutes

Ingredients:

4 cups chicken broth

1 cup low fat cream

1 teaspoon thyme dried

3 cups canned whole, peeled tomatoes

2 tablespoons almond butter

3 garlic cloves, peeled

Pepper as needed

How To:

1.   Take a stockpot and first add the butter to the bottom of a stockpot.

2.   Then add all the ingredients except heavy cream into it.

3.   Bring to a boil.

4.   Simmer for 40 minutes.

5.   Warm the heavy cream and stir into the soup.

6.   Serve and enjoy!

Nutrition (Per Serving)

Calories: 141

Fat: 12g

Carbohydrates: 4g

Protein: 4g

Chipotle Chicken Chowder

Serving: 4

Prep Time: 10 minutes

Cook Time: 23 minutes

Ingredients:

1 medium onion, chopped

2 garlic cloves, minced

6 bacon slices, chopped

4 cups jicama, cubed

3 cups chicken stock

1 teaspoon salt

2 cups low-fat, cream1 tablespoon olive oil

2 tablespoons fresh cilantro, chopped

1 ¼ pounds chicken, thigh boneless, cut into 1 inch chunks ½ teaspoon pepper

1 chipotle pepper, minced

How To:

1.   Heat olive oil over medium heat in a large sized saucepan, add bacon.

2.   Cook until crispy, add onion, garlic, and jicama.

3.   Cook for 7 minutes, add chicken stock and chicken.

4.   Bring to a boil and reduce temperature to low.

5.   Simmer for 10 minutes

6.   Season with salt and pepper.

7.   Add heavy cream and chipotle, simmer for 5 minutes.

8.   Sprinkle chopped cilantro and serve, enjoy!

Nutrition (Per Serving)

Calories: 350

Fat: 22g

Carbohydrates: 8g

Protein: 22g

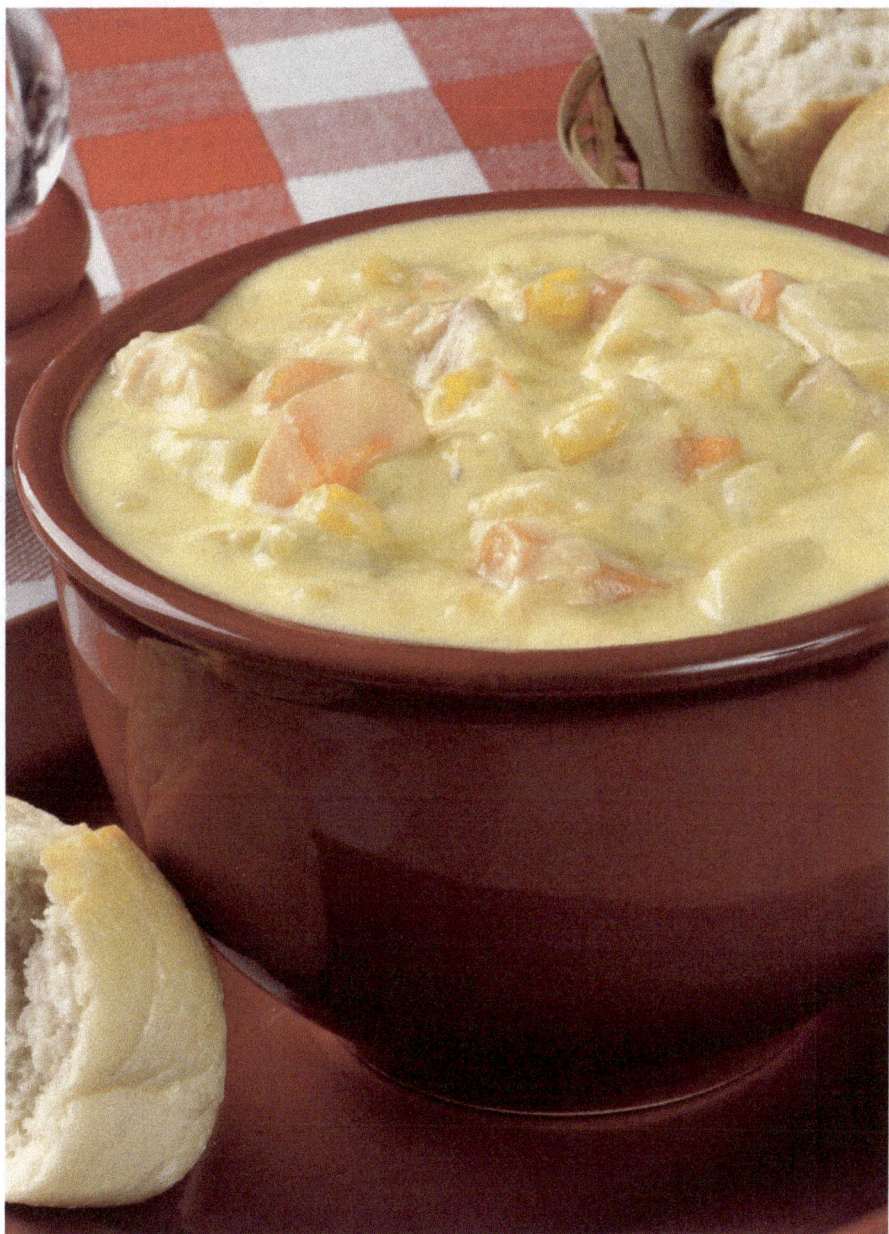

www.ingramcontent.com/pod-product-compliance
Lightning Source LLC
Chambersburg PA
CBHW050750030426
42336CB00012B/1752